PRAISE FO

IT'S

The Parent/Child Manual on Divorce

"An excellent source of divorce survival information. An invaluable aid, offering support, hope, and comfort."
—Michael S. Prokop,
author of *Divorce Happens to the Nicest Kids*

"This book provides clear and practical suggestions for dealing with real-life problems. I heartily recommend this useful resource."
—Neville L. Kyle, Ph.D., Chief of Psychological Services, the Hacker Clinic, Los Angeles

It's O.K. to Say No!

"An extremely useful book that gives lots of practical advice. The most useful and charming part of the book is a series of stories which parents can read to and then discuss with their children. The lessons are acceptable, unfrightening, and effective because they are presented in this dialogue form."
—Mrs. Louise Bates Ames, Associate Director, Gesell Institute of Human Development; author, syndicated newspaper column "Parents Ask"

"A useful resource for teachers, parents, community organizations and others concerned with educating children about protecting themselves from people who might victimize them. A sensitive, easy-to-understand approach."
—*Magazine & Bookseller*

A PARENT/CHILD MANUAL FOR THE PROTECTION OF CHILDREN

IT'S O.K. TO SAY NO TO CIGARETTES AND ALCOHOL!

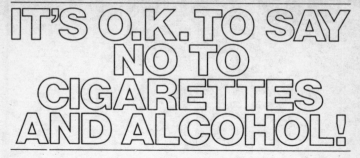

NEAL SHUSTERMAN

Illustrated by Neal Yamamoto

TOR®

A TOM DOHERTY ASSOCIATES BOOK
NEW YORK

IT'S O.K. TO SAY NO TO CIGARETTES AND ALCOHOL!

Copyright © 1988 by RGA Publishing Group, Inc.

All rights reserved, including the right to reproduce this book or
portions thereof in any form.

A TOR Book
Published by Tom Doherty Associates, Inc.
49 West 24 Street
New York, NY 10010

ISBN: 0-812-59483-5   Can. ISBN: 0-812-59484-3

Library of Congress Catalog Card Number: 88-50631

First edition: November 1988

Printed in the United States of America

0 9 8 7 6 5 4 3 2 1

Introduction

According to the American Lung Association, smoking, more than the use of all other drugs combined, will cut short the lives of today's high school students.

According to the National Council on Alcoholism, nearly one in five teenagers shows signs of developing serious alcohol problems.

We would all just as soon never see our kids smoke or drink—for their health and for our peace of mind—but studies show that kids are smoking and drinking in greater numbers and at younger ages every year. The statistics are alarming: A study done by the National Parents' Resource Institute for Drug Education (PRIDE) showed that 43% of seventh graders were already experimenting with wine and beer, and 23% with hard liquor. Another study showed that 5% of kids aged ten to thirteen get drunk at least once a week—and that number goes up to 20% in children of high school age.

The statistics on smoking are no better. A survey of adult smokers showed that two-thirds become addicted during adolescence. In 1985, one in five high school seniors was a smoker.

In and of themselves tobacco and alcohol are bad enough. We all know their frightening effects on our bodies. Smoking can lead to lung cancer, which is the cause of 25% of all cancer deaths, as well as emphysema and heart disease. Alcoholism slowly destroys the body's organs, seriously impairs the functioning of the mind, and through drunk driving, is indirectly one of the highest causes of teenage deaths.

Behind the obvious health hazards there is an underlying threat, one that demands that we give tobacco and alcohol use by

1

children even more attention. Tobacco and alcohol, the so-called "licit drugs," have become stepping-stones to much harder and even more dangerous drugs.

Chapter One
The Gateway
Drugs

Addictive behaviors are addictive behaviors, plain and simple. Chain smoking is little different from cocaine addiction when you look at the frequency as well as the psychological and physical dependency on the habit. Sure, the results and social acceptability are radically different, but the basic mechanism of addiction is the same. Once a human being takes that first step and learns his first addiction, it becomes frighteningly easy to become addicted again and again, each addiction laying the groundwork for deeper, more devastating addictions. This is the Gateway Hypothesis.

The Gateway Hypothesis states that drug abuse—just like every other undesirable behavior—begins with something readily available and somewhat socially acceptable. It begins with the "licit" drugs of tobacco and alcohol—the Gateway Drugs of addiction. From there kids proceed to hard liquor, marijuana, and then cocaine, or whatever other drugs happen to be in fashion and easily available.

Not every kid passes through that gateway. Not every kid who begins smoking becomes a drug addict, but the potential is always there, and in our era, the potential keeps growing.

It seems that innocence dies at a younger age every year. Today's nine-year-old is no more innocent than a fifteen-year-old was twenty years ago. Kids are wise to the ways of the world, and know an awful lot about things their parents probably wish they'd never heard of at all. Unfortunately, wisdom does not follow on the heels of knowledge.

3

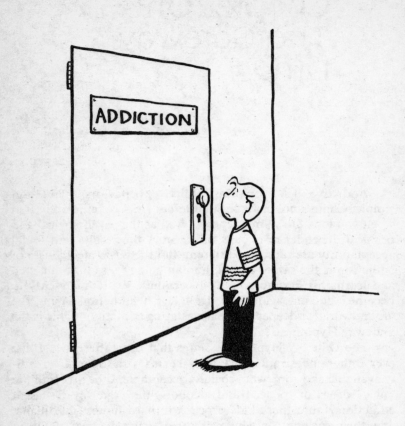

Today's ten-year-old knows how one uses cocaine, what crack is, how to smoke marijuana, and because they know so much about the drugs, their distance from them is not as great as it was for previous generations. Kids' perceptions of hard drugs move closer and closer to their perceptions of cigarettes and alcohol every day, because the other drugs are almost as commonplace. Nowadays if a child steps through the addictive gateway, he may find himself lost in a dark world, the gate shut behind him, before he gains the wisdom to turn around.

A Note on Smokeless Tobacco

Nicotine can be absorbed through the gums. Chewing tobacco is every bit as addictive as cigarettes, and is considered a gateway drug as well. On top of this, connections have been made between the use of smokeless tobacco and the development of certain forms of oral cancer. Because of all this, in August 1986, radio and television ads for smokeless tobacco were banned. Cigarette ads have been banned since January 1971. It is important that your child know that smokeless tobacco carries with it all the negative effects of cigarettes.

Also, several chewing tobacco companies are notorious for blatantly trying to attract kids to the habit. For example, they may give out free samples to young people, or sponsor tobacco-spitting contests at fairs.

Allowing your child to use smoking tobacco is on a par with giving them permission to smoke, as far as drugs are concerned.

A Note on Prevention

Studies show that children develop their attitudes towards abusable substances by the time they are ten years old.

Is it any wonder, then, that the addicted fifteen-year-old is so hard to reach? If someone had reached him or her when he or she was eight, there would be no problem now.

If lack of foresight were a disease, then our society would be infected beyond measure. We are by nature a society of "fire fighters"; we ignore a situation until there is a fire, then spend most of our time running around stomping the fire out—a fire that might be preventable, if we used foresight.

Drug abuse in today's youth is one of the most devastating and uncontrollable of these blazes, and often it seems that all our efforts to douse the flames have the effect of a garden hose against a forest fire.

Prevention, psychologists and educators agree, is the most effective way to fight drug abuse. There are three very important points to note:

a) Prevention must begin in the home.

b) Prevention must begin before a child's attitudes are set (in other words, before a child is ten).

c) Prevention must not only address hard drugs but should also deal with the drugs that lead up to them, namely, tobacco and alcohol.

With all this in mind, this book is designed as an effective preventive medicine against drug abuse. It will help you and your child, through the strength of your own relationship, develop methods of combating the pressure to begin drinking or smoking, and in so doing, will ward off the use of harder drugs.

We'll begin with a look at some of the different environments kids are raised in today, and what behavior to expect from children in each type of household.

Chapter Two
The Home Environment

Every home is different, every family has different values, and for every home there are special considerations that have to be taken into account when determining how the home environment will influence a child.

What follows are brief descriptions of several different types of households, and how they might affect youngsters in relation to tobacco and alcohol. Keep in mind that these are generalizations—many households may fall into more than one of the categories listed below, and some of the categories can easily overlap.

The Moderate-Drinking/Non-Smoking Household

. . . in which drinking, usually of beer or wine, is an occasional, but not regular, occurrence. The adults don't drink to get drunk, or to wind down. They drink probably for the same reason they eat cheesecake; the alcohol is there, they enjoy the feelings it provokes, and there's a commercial on the TV. In other words,

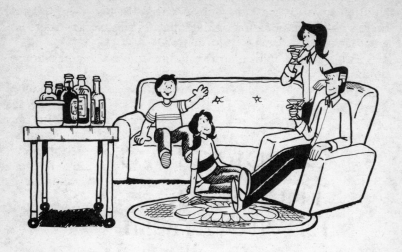

drinking is not special, "adult" behavior, it's not a big deal, and it's not something that's particularly desirable. Included in this classification are households where it is culturally permissible for children as well as adults to drink wine at meals.

Children raised in this environment will not feel that there is any mystique about alcohol. Assuming that their personality development is up to par, and that they've learned how to say "No" to peer pressure, they will have no psychological predispositions to drinking.

Studies show that children who are introduced to moderate alcohol by their families tend to begin drinking during their teenage years, frequently in the presence of their parents. They usually do *not* develop alcoholism. These parents have self-regulatory habits that their children learn. In this type of home, a teenager knows when to stop.

The Cloistered Household

. . . is the other side of the coin. This family does its best to shield children from the evils of the world by covering their eyes. Some parents think that if they don't talk about something, that thing does not exist. They believe that if they censor their children's world, the kids will be safe from bad things. Thus, there's no communication on the topic of drug use, and there is a great lack of trustworthy information.

Two types of child tend to emerge from a cloistered household:

The rebel. Normal adolescent rebellion becomes much more powerful, because there is a strong need to get out of the "cloister." A kid who jumps from a cloistered household may never be able to come back; often they jump as far as they can go. This is the classic self-destructive child from a good home.

The successfully cloistered child. This child has never been allowed to develop much of a personality, and usually lacks socializing skills as well.

The Smoking Household

. . . in which at least one adult in the family smokes. Here's a documented fact: 75% of all teenage smokers come from families where one or both parents smoke. If you or your spouse smokes, don't be too surprised if your children start smoking, because you're setting the example. Telling them not to smoke is a case of "Do as I say, not as I do," which is the weakest argument to use with any child. This tack will blow a good deal of your credibility.

If you enjoy smoking, and your child knows it, the chances are higher that he or she will smoke. If you smoke, but you really want to quit, you might be able to make him or her realize that you've got·a problem he or she can avoid.

Far and away, the best way to keep your child from smoking is to not smoke yourself. This may not be what you want to hear, but it's the truth. Don't expect any person or any book to come up with a way to keep your child away from cigarettes if you can't.

On the other hand, a friend of mine, as a child, would continually flush his mother's cigarettes down the toilet. (As I recall, he had problems sitting down because he got spanked so much.) The point is, some kids may react violently to cigarette smoke even if they've had to put up with it all their lives. If your

9

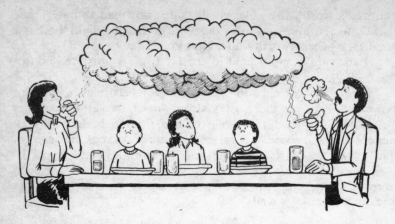

kids are militant non-smokers now, and make you miserable every time you light up, chances are they'll be just as much against smoking when they grow up—how else could they teach you a lesson!

(Incidentally, my friend finally won; his mother quit smoking. Now he's married, and is continually flushing his wife's cigarettes. I believe he still gets spanked.)

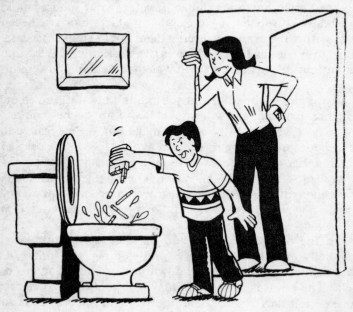

The Recreational-Drinking Household

. . . in which drinking is acceptable when the adults want to have a good time. This is a common type of household. Children in recreational-drinking homes tend to connect alcohol with good times and friends. Thus, in adolescence, and maybe even before, these children may choose to drink with friends to be social.

If you catch them, and raise a stink, they will probably resent you because, after all, they are just imitating you. "But *you* do it," says Cindy, to which her mother or father invariably replies, "Well, we're adults."

Cindy hates that, because it implies that she is a child. It also implies that drinking is an adult thing to do, which is one of the primary reasons why kids begin drinking: they want to be adult.

What a parent means when he or she says, "Well, we're adults," is, "You haven't lived enough to deal with what alcohol can do to you. You don't have enough perspective on life to drink."

Of course, if her mother or father told Cindy that, she'd still be as frustrated, because life experience is something she can't buy, no matter how large her allowance—but at least the honest answer would make her think.

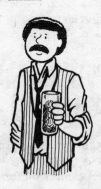

If recreational drinking is an accepted part of life in your home, that's fine; after all, most of us do drink recreationally every now and again—but keep an eye on your kids, because they *are* at risk.

The Alcohol-as-Stress-Relief Household

. . . where it is acceptable and commonplace for the adult members of the household to relax with a drink, to use alcohol to calm their nerves. No one in the house is truly an alcoholic, but alcohol does serve a specific function that the child can easily perceive. Little Peter sees his daddy come home from work every day and have a drink, and learns that when Daddy feels tense or under stress, Daddy needs a drink. Therefore Peter learns that drinking makes Daddy feel better.

By age ten, alcohol is part of Peter's permanent code of values, registered as an acceptable form of stress relief. In adolescence, when anxiety attacks from all directions with kamikaze accuracy, Peter may suddenly realize or decide that he needs a drink. How far he will go depends on how much anxiety he is experiencing, how much self-control he has, and how many other methods of stress relief he has learned.

In this type of household it is important to help the child develop other forms of stress relief—perhaps jogging, or swimming, or some other sport, providing the emphasis is on enjoyment, not competition.

The Alcoholic Household

. . . where at least one adult member of the household is an alcoholic. This is always a traumatic experience. Perhaps nowhere else can a child get a clearer picture of how addiction can devastate human beings. Unfortunately, in the alcoholic household the child is one of the human beings who are being emotionally and psychologically devastated.

Studies show that children of alcoholics tend to—at first—stay away from alcohol, but when they experience stress in their adult lives, alcoholism and other addictive behaviors may emerge. Because the alcoholic household has such a long-term effect on children, it is very dangerous. Most methods intended to prevent childhood use of alcohol are designed to carry children through their teen years, until they have the perspective to make responsible decisions. This assumes, however, that their personalities have not been damaged, and there is no telling what damage an alcoholic household can cause.

The Drug-Permissive Household

In our society, marijuana is becoming as accepted a drug as alcohol. A certain kind of marijuana-using household could be more accurately classified between the recreational-drinking home and the alcoholic home, for it may not be as dysfunctional as an alcoholic household. To avoid making a black-and-white distinction on a blurred line of social acceptability, let's define the drug-permissive household as one in which drug use extends beyond mild use of marijuana.

The drug-permissive household, in which the attitude toward and use of the various illicit drugs is very casual, is the household in which children are most at risk. If a child is raised around drugs, and his or her parents suddenly turn around and tell him or her not to smoke or drink, the child will probably laugh in the parents' faces and do what ever he or she damn well pleases.

The message behind this whole chapter is something you should already know. *You* are your child's primary role model. Picture your child at the age of twenty. You should be *now* what you want your child to be *then*. There's nothing wrong with a recreational-drinking household, or a smoking household—if you don't mind your kids smoking or drinking recreationally.

Other Factors

Here's a checklist of other elements of home life that can affect a child's choice to begin using the gateway drugs.

What Is Your Child Like?

Is your child a television addict?

It has been suggested that there is a parallel between the passivity of "television addiction" and the passivity of a drug high. Television should not fill too great a place in your child's life. Encourage him or her in activities other than watching television.

Does your child have too many toys?

When children continually receive new toys, they often become bored very quickly. As a child gets older, the door is open for addictive substances to be used to alleviate that boredom.

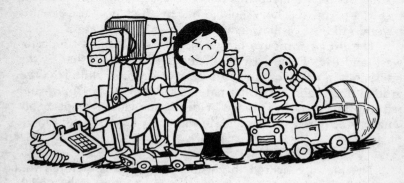

Is your child easily frustrated?

Children who tend to be easily frustrated may tend to give up in troubled times, and may give in to addictive substances as they get older.

What Sort of Parent Are You?

Do you expect too much from your child?

Modern kids have a great deal of stress put on them by school, sports, peer pressure, themselves, and even by you. It's rare to find a stress-free child, or a stress-free adult for that matter, but you can lower the level of stress in your child by not pushing too hard.

For instance, if Wesley Junior is not an "A" student, and Wesley Senior was, that's life; his father must learn to accept it. Expecting your children to be something they're not is exactly the sort of stress that leads to emergency "solutions." Alcohol is one of those easy "solutions" that is not a solution at all.

It's important to help your children set goals, but always make sure that these goals, whether set by parents or children, are realistic and attainable.

Competitive sports is another area where kids develop high levels of stress. It's fine to be competitive, as long as children don't feel they have to win at all costs.

Do you over-indulge your child?

Children who are "spoiled" learn that they can have everything they want with no effort. When things suddenly don't come so easily, they become frustrated, and seek quick ways of gratifying themselves. This gratification may begin with alcohol, then spread to harder drugs.

Are you an "authoritarian" parent?

An *authoritarian* household is one where the parents "lay down the law" with a dogmatic iron fist, regardless of children's feelings or opinions. The word of the authoritarian parent is the indisputable word of God. When it comes to drug abuse, it has been determined that this type of parenting *is every bit as dangerous as a parent who does not supervise a child.*

On the other hand, an *authoritative* household is one in which parents provide rules but are sensitive to their children's needs, feelings, and opinions.

The authoritative household, in which parental authority provides a sense of security for children, also provides a basis for a child's own self-esteem. The children of these homes are less likely to begin smoking or heavy drinking.

Is there a history of alcoholism in your family?

It has recently come to light that biological factors can affect a person's response to addictive substances. In short, there is evidence to show that alcoholism, in some cases, may be hereditary. One study, of adopted children, showed that biological sons of alcoholic fathers were three times more likely to become alcoholics themselves, and new test results are coming to light every day.

These studies show that a predisposition to addiction can be passed from parent to child. It is biologically much easier for these people to become alcoholics. The smallest amount of alcohol can lead to an addiction.

It is also easy for such people to become addicted to other substances, such as cocaine. If you suspect that you, and consequently your child, may have a biological predisposition to addiction, contact a physician for advice.

Chapter Three
Keys to Prevention

Preventing substance abuse five years before you expect it to happen is a touchy business. You never quite know if you've "done the right thing" until you see how your kid handles adolescence. If your child comes through without having gone off the deep end, you can assume that either you did all the right things, or you were very lucky.

Although there appears to be a great deal of guesswork involved in child-raising, that's not really the case. Once you understand how kids from even the best of backgrounds can slip into substance abuse, half the battle is won. Once you understand, you have the tools to help your kids.

There are countless complex reasons for every type of behavior—the entire science of psychology is based on navigating the infinite maze of human behavior. Rather than concerning ourselves with psychology, let's focus on three facets of a child's life that most effectively guide his or her development: perception, personality development, and parent-child relationships.

Perception

Beauty is in the eye of the beholder. One man's meat is another man's poison. Dozens of maxims attest to the fact that no two people perceive the same thing in the same way. Children are no different. They are born into a confusing world of light and motion. They must learn the meaning of everything they see. They must learn the rules of acceptable behavior. Children are bombarded by millions of bits of information every second, from a myriad of sources: the media, including television, radio, film, and all forms of advertising; as well as more personal sources, such as parents, siblings, and peers.

In growing up, children must learn to decide for themselves what is important and what's not. For instance, three children seeing a cigarette advertisement on a billboard may see and remember different things from it. Ben notices the happy, smiling people with cigarettes and subconsciously notes that good-looking, rich, happy people smoke. Julie sees the surgeon general's warning, and subconsciously concludes that if smoking needs a warning, it must really be bad for you. Edwin might not even remember the smiling smokers, or the surgeon general's warning, because he was too busy looking at the huge steel frame of the billboard, wondering whether or not it would fall down in an earthquake. Every child perceives things differently.

Psychologists say that the mind is like a black box. Information goes in, sits in the black box for a while, and comes out as a response. No one knows what goes on in the black box. Behavioral psychology is based on the idea that the internal process

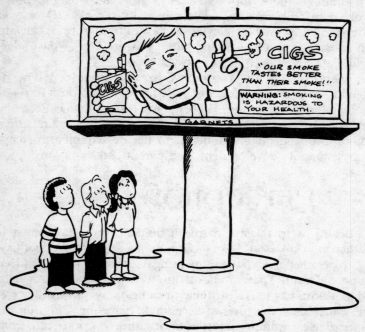

doesn't matter, as long as you get the required response. Unfortunately, by the time we get a response from a teenager's "black box," it's too late to change the nature of the information being assessed.

Therefore it is important to have some idea of how your child perceives the world. The best way to get a glimpse into your children's perceptions is to watch them, talk to them, and listen to them.

Here's a list of the various ideas children develop about cigarettes and alcohol:

Alcohol is relaxing.
Alcohol is for good times.
Alcohol is grown-up.
Alcohol makes you feel good.
Alcohol is like a magical potion.
Only smart people drink.
Rich people smoke.
Fancy people drink hard liquor.
Cool people smoke.
Everybody drinks at weddings.
Good Americans drink beer.
Drinking makes you forget your problems.
Real men get drunk.
You're a nerd if you don't smoke.
The more you smoke, the more you like it.
It's easy to quit.
You have more friends if you smoke.
College is one big beer party.
Smoking and drinking impress others.
Famous people always smoke and drink.
Alcohol is an acquired taste.
Drunk people are fun and funny.
Smoking helps you lose weight.

Here's a list of the anti-cigarette and anti-alcohol messages they should be getting, either from outside sources or from you:

You can't think right when you drink.
Beer can make you fat.
Drinking makes you feel sick.

Smoking makes your clothes and hair smell bad.
Drunks look like idiots.
Drunk driving can kill you.
Smoking hurts your lungs.
Smoking turns your teeth yellow.
Smoking gives you bad breath.
Smoking makes it hard to breathe.
Smoking is inconsiderate to those around you.
Drinking makes you forget things.
Drinking makes you talk funny.
Cigarettes and alcohol cost lots of money.
Once you start, it's hard to stop.
Smoking causes cancer.
Drinking too much can kill you.

It is important to note that for very young children, the more immediate the effect, the easier it is for them to understand. Telling a young boy or girl, "Smoking makes your clothes smell bad," may have a stronger effect than telling him or her that it causes cancer.

Personality Development

By the time a child reaches adolescence, the structure of his or her personality has been set. The home life of the pre-adolescent provides the building blocks for personality. If you give a child Tinkertoys to work with, chances are the stress tests of adolescence will take a heavy toll.

There are many different schools of thought on parental involvement in the development of their children's personalities, but all agree that parents are the most important influence on a developing personality. Though you may at times feel helpless in raising your children, you aren't. If you've done a good job, the values you have taught and the strengths you have helped your child develop will always be somewhere at the core of his or her personality, even during the difficult, rebellious years.

In addition to a personal code of ethics, decision-making skills and self-esteem are highly important to a developing child. This is why it is important to help your children build confidence in themselves and their own decisions.

It's a natural tendency for parents to want to control the lives of young children, because control means protection. You review their teachers, you approve their friends, you decide your children's daily schedule. Many times, however, this type of control goes too far, and becomes damaging to your child. Here's a brief checklist to see if you're hindering the development of decision-making skills in your child.

Do you tend to make all your children's decisions for them?
Do you ask for your child's opinion?
When you do hear his or her opinion, do you take it seriously or not?
Do you insist that you're always right, and when you're wrong, do you avoid admitting it to your child?

Self-esteem goes hand in hand with decision-making skills. Adults are also notorious for knocking down a child's self-esteem without realizing it.

Do you ever say, "I told you so," when your child fails at something or makes a mistake?
Do you often forget to congratulate your child for a job well done?
Do you often point out the negatives to your child, rather than praise the positives?
Do you scoff at things your child finds very important?

Penny is a child raised in such an environment. She has learned that her opinions are worthless, her decisions are invalid, and her feelings are silly. When she emerges from the parental iron grip, she becomes a compulsive follower, unable to stand up for her own thoughts and feelings. She is at the mercy of whatever group she ends up following.

Children have to be allowed to make decisions at an early age. True, you know better than your child when it comes to many things, but it is important to allow him or her to come to his or her own conclusions, rather than forcing him or her to accept your conclusions. Unless there is danger or great inconvenience involved, it's better to allow a child to learn from his or her mistakes. Don't try to "save him the trouble." All you'll "save him" is the valuable experience every decision brings.

Here are two interactions concerning the same subject. One builds decision-making skills, one damages them.

WRONG	RIGHT
KEVIN: From now on I'm going to do my homework after my favorite TV show, instead of before.	KEVIN: From now on I'm going to do my homework after my favorite TV show, instead of before.
DAD: That's stupid, you'll never get it done.	DAD: Will you get it all done?
THE NEXT DAY:	KEVIN: Sure I will.
KEVIN: Dad, I'm too tired to finish my homework.	THE NEXT DAY:
DAD: I told you so, but no, you didn't listen. Now you'll have to get up early tomorrow and do it.	KEVIN: Dad, I'm too tired to finish my homework.
	DAD: Then you'll have to wake up early and finish it before school.
	KEVIN: I think I'll go back to doing it before I watch TV.

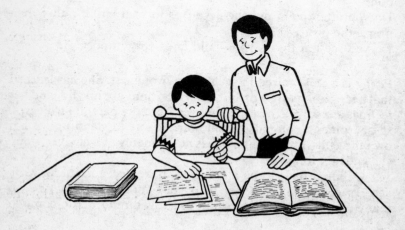

22

The best way to test whether or not your children are learning the values you've been teaching is to allow them to make their own decisions whenever possible. On the occasions where you have to put your foot down, always give a rational, sensible reason for your answer:

MOM: No, you can't stay outside in the rain.
JENNY: Why not?
MOM: Because it's cold and you just got over the flu.

If you ever feel tempted to say, "Because I said so," keep in mind that, though this can be effective with very young children, it is not only annoying but completely unhelpful for an older child. This response, when given consistently, teaches a poor pattern of making decisions and dealing with others.

Giving your child the logical reason, even if he or she still protests your decision, teaches him or her that there is a good reason for everything you say—that your decisions are not made on random whims. It teaches a child that decisions are grounded in knowledge. Provide that knowledge, and the necessary explanations, to your children, and their decisions will be rational and sensible.

Parent-Child Relationships

Because parents are so important in children's perceptions and in their personality development, parent-child relationships are of paramount importance.

Unfortunately, these relationships are undermined by today's society. Kids spend more time with peers, or away from home in after-school programs. Many families are single-parent households, and often, when there are two parents, both work. When families are together, television, movies, and countless other forms of entertainment take the place of family interaction.

Keeping a foothold in a child's development used to be a natural consequence of family life. It's not anymore. Paying the rent and keeping your children clothed and fed is no longer enough. There needs to be active communication. You need to be an active participant in your children's lives. This could be as simple as playing a game with them one night, instead of sitting passively in front of the television. Just talking is always helpful.

The key is not time, but *quality time*. It's not always easy to be there for our children when our own lives are so hectic—so we have to make a conscious effort to *be* there, in mind as well as body. Communication is the key.

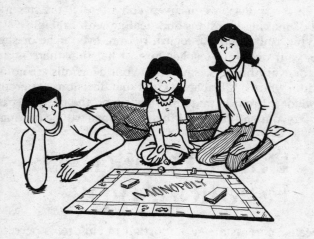

Chapter Four
The Media

The media have developed an increasingly solid stance against drug use; however, their treatment of alcohol and cigarettes is incredibly inconsistent. After all, alcohol and cigarettes are an accepted part of life, yet as more and more youngsters become alcoholics, as more and more kids pass beyond the gateway drugs, the more that responsible adults realize something has to be done. Thus the media produce a whirlwind of ambivalence that can't help but confuse our kids.

Take television, for example. One moment there's a commercial against drunk driving. Next there's a smiling "party animal" dog, and beautiful women singing the praises of lite beer. One moment the queens of prime-time television smoke cigarettes in sequined dresses, then the haunting image of Yul Brynner appears, telling us that he died of lung cancer because he smoked. These messages are clear to adults who have already made their peace with cigarettes and alcohol—but kids have not made their decisions. Who knows how the media are affecting their perceptions?

Advertisements are most effective on a passive, accepting audience. Once you see behind the motives of advertisements, they become less effective. Children watching a beer commercial may not have considered anything beyond the fact that the people in the commercial seem to be having a good time. It becomes your task to enlighten them in this area, something done most effectively while the commercial is still fresh in their memories. In this example, Rhonda and her father are watching TV together when a beer commercial comes on.

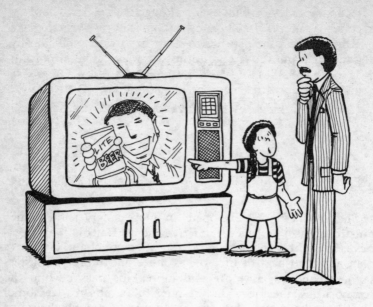

DAD (POINTING AT THE SET): Who is that guy?

RHONDA: You know him, that's that famous comedian.

DAD: How about the rest of the people in the bar?

RHONDA: I don't know. They look like surfers.

DAD: You think they really are?

RHONDA: They're just actors, I guess.

DAD: Do you think he really likes that beer?

RHONDA: I guess so.

DAD: I heard he gets paid close to a million dollars to make these commercials!

RHONDA: A million dollars? Just to talk about beer? Where do they get all that money?

DAD: From the beer they sell. (Rhonda nods.) Why do you think all these people look so happy?

RHONDA: Because they get paid to.

DAD: Who pays them?

RHONDA: The company that makes the beer?

DAD: That's right. Why do you think they do that?

RHONDA: To sell more beer. Boy, that sure is a cheap trick.

It's a simple lesson that every kid needs to learn. There's a good chance your kid already knows it, but it never hurts to make sure. Rhonda's dad helped her to draw her own conclusion by asking the right questions and not lecturing her. The important thing is to get the child interested in the conversation. Otherwise you might end up with responses like "Yeah," "I don't know," and "Oh," which usually indicates that the child isn't thinking at all, and the conversation will take a hasty flight out of the other ear the second you're not looking.

On the negative side of conversations like these is the implied message that drinking will make you rich and famous. It's important that your children understand that this isn't true—it's what the advertiser would like them to believe.

As far as television commercials go, there are two more points that will give your child something to think about. A) cigarette commercials have been banned from television, and B) one cannot drink alcohol on a commercial—and if television doesn't allow something, there may be a good reason for it.

We've talked about the indirect influences of the media, things kids happen to pick up in passing, messages that were generally not meant for them. Far more important are the elements of the media that are directly geared toward them. Early evening television programs, popular music, music videos, and a significant portion of feature films are geared toward a youthful audience.

Because of the huge amount of money the youth market brings, the media have a tendency to pander to that audience, showing kids whatever they will pay money to see.

We can't control what goes into our children's eyes and ears. Groups across the country fight to ban songs from the radio, or to pull magazines from the shelves, to mixed effect. That type of censorship is frightening, however, because there are always those who will take it to book-burning extremes. The truth is that censorship of this type has the opposite effect. The more parents want something censored, the more enticing it becomes. That's human nature.

Clearly the secret is not to close kids' eyes to world, but to open them far enough to allow children to sift through the mixed messages given by the media. Rather than turning off the lights in the maze, we must help them find their way through it.

Among the biggest culprits in directing pro-alcohol and pro-cigarette messages at children are music videos. You can discourage your kids from watching such things, as many parents do, but chances are, they'll still see their fair share.

Just as with commercials, if a kid understands the motivation behind pro-cigarette or pro-alcohol messages in entertainment, he or she is better equipped to judge them.

MOM: You like this video?

MATTHEW: It's rad. See this part? Here's where he eats a rat, and then drowns in a bathtub filled with vodka, while smoking fifteen cigarettes.

MOM: That guy sure has a wild act. You think he does it for real or just for show?

MATTHEW: For show, I guess. I heard that in real life, he's very quiet. There's some rock stars who really act crazy all the time, though.

MOM: And lots of rock stars have miserable lives. Which ones do you think are like that?

MATTHEW: Probably the ones who act crazy in real life. You know, the ones who drink a lot and do drugs.

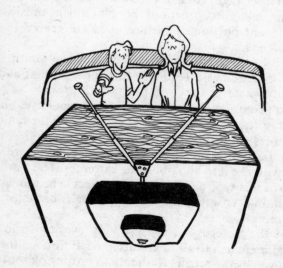

You may not be able to stop your children from watching questionable videos, but you can help give them a healthier perception of what they're looking at.

Chapter Five
Taking the Offensive: Teaching Your Child to Say No

Thus far this book has dealt with a defense against the use of tobacco and alcohol, but a strong offense is also needed. In other words, it is important to A) actively teach your child the facts about tobacco and alcohol, and B) teach your child how to stay away from tobacco and alcohol.

Studies show that frightening kids away from drugs simply doesn't work. "Social inoculation" programs—which teach children specific ways of responding to pressure situations—have been shown to be the most effective way of keeping kids away from drugs. The "Say No" strategy is social inoculation, and therefore, teaching our kids to say no is one of the strongest weapons we have against the gateway drugs. Parental support, communication, and decision-making skills are highly important, but if a child can't refuse a friend who offers him or her a drink, the rest doesn't matter.

Keep in mind that the term "social inoculation" does not imply that there's a "vaccine" against the gateway drugs. No child is ever immune, but it is possible to instill a higher resistance in your child.

The first step in teaching your children about cigarettes and alcohol is to find out what they think, and what they know. Here are a few actual discussions I had with kids about cigarettes and alcohol.

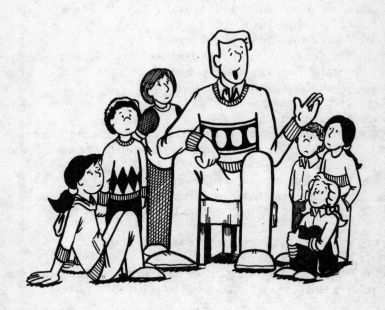

All these conversations took place at a summer day camp, in a public park, with children who knew me and felt comfortable talking with me. Each conversation was started by me making an offhand comment about an empty beer bottle or cigarette butt, of which there are no shortages in public parks. After that I found most kids were very willing to give their opinions.

NEAL: What do you think about cigarettes?

MIKE (AGE SEVEN): They're disgusting, they're bad for your lungs, and they give you cancer.

NEAL: What makes cigarettes bad?

MIKE: I don't know.

NEAL: What's alcohol?

MIKE: I don't know. That's the bad stuff in beer, isn't it?

JULIE (AGE EIGHT): My mom got divorced because my dad smoked. Well, that, and he did drugs too. One time I was at a restaurant when I was four, and they gave me a little straw to drink with and I said, "Oh, Daddy uses that kind of straw for his drugs."

NEAL: What do you think about drugs?

JULIE: They're awful for you. Drugs make you wild and mess up your brain. They can make you die.

NEAL: What about alcohol?

JULIE: That's a drug too.

NEAL: And cigarettes?

JULIE: They don't make you wild, but you can die from them.

NEAL: What would you do if someone came up to you and offered you a cigarette?

JULIE: I would say no and walk away.

NEAL: What if it were your best friend?

JULIE: I would say, "I don't need a friend that does that."

JOEY (AGE FIVE): Are cigarettes the same as drugs?

NEAL: What do you think?

JOEY: Well, I think that cigarettes have drugs in them, because you get stuck on cigarettes like you get stuck on drugs.

NEAL: What's a cigarette?

CODY (AGE FIVE): That's something people smoke on and they can die on it.

NEAL: Why can they die?

CODY: Because smoke can turn into fire inside you.

NEAL: Where inside you?

CODY: Your stomach.

NEAL: Do your parents smoke?

CODY: No, and I'm glad, because I don't want them to die too soon.

NEAL: What's alcohol?

CODY: Something if you drink you can get dead and die.

NEAL: What has alcohol in it?

CODY: Beer. I think that's all.

NEAL: What is that?

SHARON (AGE SEVEN): It's a cigarette.

NEAL: Do your parents smoke?

SHARON: No, but my father used to.

NEAL: Are you glad that your father quit?

SHARON: Yes, because smoking's bad for you; it can cause cancer, and it's bad for your lungs.

NEAL: What else can happen to you if you smoke?

SHARON: You can become addicted to it; it's like a drug, or like a food that you really like, like chips—you can't stop eating them. But it's much worse with cigarettes.

RICH (AGE SIX): Cigarettes make your lungs black.

JON (AGE FIVE): When I see people smoking I feel sad.

NEAL: Why?

JON: Because they're going to die. I don't want to smoke and die.

RICH: My mom smokes. I wish she would stop.

NEAL: If smoking is so bad, then why do people do it?

JON: Because after a while they like it.

BARRY (AGE SEVEN): They become addicted.

RICH: No, they don't! They just do it because they want to. They don't care about their health and stuff.

BARRY: You do *too* get addicted!

RICH: No! My mom smokes all the time and she's not addicted.

NEAL: How do you know she's not?

RICH: Because she told me she's not.

NEAL: How about alcohol? What's that?

BARRY: It's the stuff in rum and wine, and it's bad for you.

JON: You'll die if you drink a lot of it.

BARRY: No, you won't.

RICH: You'll die if you drink rubbing alcohol, though.

JON: Yeah. Yeah, that's what I meant.

NEAL: But what about the stuff in beer and wine?

BARRY: Well, I guess you *can* die from it, but not right away.

NEAL: Why do you think adults don't want kids to drink alcohol?

RICH: Because they don't want you to die early.

JON: And they don't want you to get used to it.

BARRY: You get addicted.

RICH: Yeah, and if you're like that as a kid, you'll be really screwed up when you get older.

BARRY: *If* you get older.

NEAL: Pretend I'm an alien from another planet, and I see these smoking white sticks in people's mouths. What are those things?

MARIE (AGE EIGHT): Cigarettes.

NEAL: What's in them?

MARIE: Yucky stuff.

NEAL: What kind of yucky stuff?

MARIE: Alcohol. Cigarettes have alcohol and alcohol is bad for your lungs.

NEAL: Does anyone in your family smoke?

JASON (AGE NINE): Yeah, my mom.

NEAL: Why does she smoke?

JASON: Because she's really nervous. She tried to quit, but she's too nervous.

NEAL: Do you want her to quit?

JASON: Yeah, but not if it makes her nervous. Anyway it's okay. It's not hurting her lungs.

34

NEAL: How do you know that?

JASON: Because the doctor said so. Only *some* people get hurt lungs from smoking. All the tests show that it doesn't really hurt your lungs that much. At least most people's.

NEAL: Do you think you'll ever smoke?

JASON: Probably not. My mom gave me a cigarette to smoke once and I coughed, because my lungs are too small, but when I get older, I'd be able to take it.

As you can see, kids have different perceptions of cigarettes and alcohol; they may be more knowledgeable than you think, or be filled with misconceptions, and you won't know until you ask them.

Hearing what your kids have to say lets you know where to go from there. If your child has accurate perceptions, you can reinforce them. If his or her perceptions are erroneous, you can straighten them out.

Though your child is exposed to pro-alcohol, pro-tobacco messages every day, you have the ability to counter them. For every erroneous message, there is a truth:

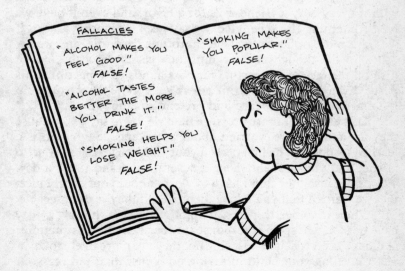

"Alcohol makes you feel good."—The truth is, it doesn't make you feel good, it makes you feel numb. In the long run, it makes you feel bad because people get violently ill and have horrible hangovers.

"Alcohol tastes better the more you drink it." In other words, the more you drink it, the harder it is to stop drinking, because you get addicted.

"Smoking helps you lose weight." Wrong! A healthy diet and exercise help you lose weight. You don't need cigarettes to control your appetite.

"Smoking makes you popular." What's popular about bad breath and yellow teeth?

Refer back to the section on perception for a more extensive list of messages you can give your child.

Saying No

Saying no is a difficult thing to do. As adults we are faced with it every day. A friend asks for a favor, and even though we have something else scheduled, we say yes. Our mother asks us if we want more of her special zucchini-tuna casserole, and we say "sure," even though her zucchini-tuna casserole is the foulest dish on the face of the earth. Our boss hands us a martini at his party. Even if you don't drink, there's a good chance you'll sip the martini in his presence and pretend to enjoy it.

Kids are under more pressure than we are to say yes, because they are much more worried about acceptance. Saying no is a learned response. The first person your children learn to say no to is you, and you probably hear it several thousand times a day. This is because they don't have to worry about your acceptance; they've learned that you'll love them even if they're disagreeable.

When it comes to peers, it's not as easy. If, however, they have been taught specific responses to specific types of situations, and have been coached in saying no, they are more likely to do it.

Coaching your child in saying no is just that: putting your child in hypothetical situations and having them say "No!" loudly, clearly, and most importantly, proudly.

Here's some things to keep in mind when teaching your child to say no:

Saying no is always more effective when there's a reason.

"Try this cigarette."
"No, it tastes bad."

"Let's drink some rum."
"No, it's bad for you."

"Want a beer?"
"No, I'll get in trouble."

Teach your child to get away from kids pressuring them to smoke or drink. The faster your child gets away from the situation, the better.

"Hey, kid . . . wanna smoke?"
"Nope. Gotta go, I'm late for school."

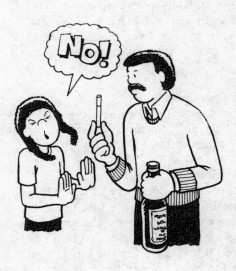

Kids often get into cigarettes and alcohol, and subsequently harder drugs, because they can't come up with anything better to do. If your child is in a situation where a friend is suggesting smoking or drinking, teach your child to offer alternatives.

"Let's drink my dad's beer."
"Naah, let's ride bikes instead."

"Let's try my mom's clove cigarettes—they smell good."
"Naah, why don't we go to the arcade?"

"Vodka makes you feel good. Let's drink some."
"Why don't we make chocolate shakes? I'll bet they make you feel better!"

Here's a list of rules of thumb when it comes to teaching your child to say no.

1) Get your child interested.
If your child is completely unreceptive, don't force the issue; they won't be listening. Usually, when a kid is in a talking mood, you can guide the conversation to any topic you wish. If your child is still unwilling to talk with you, perhaps making it into a game would help.

2) Don't burn your child out.
Kids' attention spans are notoriously short. If your child is interested in "say-no" coaching for fifteen minutes, then it should last for fifteen minutes, and no longer.

3) Once is not enough.
One session of coaching does very little. Coaching is something that should continue. Perhaps the first few sessions need to be longer, but once your child has got the idea, "booster sessions" should become a matter of course, and don't need to be of any great length. You'll find that after the initial sessions, opportunities will arise for brief spur-of-the-moment sessions that will serve as effective reminders.

LAUREN: Look at those kids over there, Dad, they're smoking!

DAD: Do they go to your school?

LAUREN: Yeah, I know them.

DAD: What would you do if one of them offered you a cigarette?

LAUREN: I'd tell her no.

DAD: But what if it was your best friend?

LAUREN: You mean Melissa?

DAD: Yes. What if Melissa gave you a cigarette?

LAUREN: I'd still tell her no.

DAD: But what if you were with all of your friends and they were all smoking?

LAUREN: I don't care, I'd tell them they were all stupid for smoking.

DAD: And what if she said she wouldn't be your friend anymore if you didn't smoke?

LAUREN: I'd tell her I don't need a friend who smokes.

A simple, unforced conversation at an appropriate time is just the sort of "booster shot" a social inoculation program needs. You may just find your child will come back to you a year down the line, saying, "Hey, remember the time you asked me what I would do if Melissa offered me a cigarette? Well, guess what?"

4) Keep your child's developmental level in mind.

Lots of parents can't communicate well with their kids, because they either talk above their kids' heads, or talk in such a condescending manner that the child can't take them seriously. It's important to judge where your child's "head is at." If your child is a wide-eyed, trusting innocent (perhaps a five- through seven-year-old), make sure he or she understands what you are saying. Have him or her explain it to you in his or her own words. If your child is slightly older, or more precocious, relate to the child on a higher level. Kids are getting sharper and more cynical at earlier ages. If they feel you're speaking down to them, they'll fold their arms and treat you with aloof cynicism until you go away.

5) Prepare your child for a variety of situations.

There are lots of situations that can lead kids into smoking or drinking, anything from pressure from a best friend to pressure from a bully. The more types of situations you can throw at your child, to help him or her think and practice saying no, the more resistance your child will build up.

I know a father and son who had a game going with each other. Each day the father would come up with a situation involving drug pressure, and the child had to come up with a clever way of saying no and getting out of it.

The kid turned out to be quite vocal in his school when it came to cigarettes and alcohol, and he was a formidable opponent for anyone who offered him a smoke or a drink.

When saying no becomes a natural, matter-of-course response, then, if the real situation arises, saying no should not be difficult.

6) Let your kids know that they're not alone.
Kids get into cigarettes and alcohol to be with the "in group." Once they know that there's another group of kids—the better "in" group—who have learned to say no, it becomes easier to say it. Joining an organized support group, or getting together informally with some other concerned families, can help you and your child create positive bonds, and will help your child feel less isolated in pressure situations.

A Few Words On Two-Way Communication

MOM (SHOUTING): I don't want you doing that anymore, do you understand me?
PETER: (wide-eyed nod).
MOM (SHOUTING): It was stupid! You could have hurt somebody! Do you understand me?
PETER: (wide-eyed nod).
MOM: You should know better! How many times do I have to tell you? How many? Do you hear me?
PETER: (wide-eyed nod).
MOM: Are you going to do it again?
PETER: (wide-eyed nod).

Every parent has experienced a situation like this. Needless to say, it is not the best form of communication. A lecture is a one-way monologue. The child is forced to listen, or to pretend to listen. If you're angry, they may not hear you because they're worrying about what will happen when you're done talking. Will they be spanked? Will they lose TV privileges?

Sometimes kids just "check out" and think of something else entirely—dinner or a baseball game—while still giving you perfunctory yeses and noes until you're satisfied.

Communication implies two-way interaction: you speak and your child responds. It is important to elicit intelligent responses from children—responses they have to think about.

Here's a conversation that might take place in a household where the father is an alcoholic.

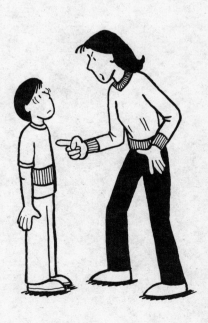

MOM: Why did you drink Daddy's scotch?

STEPHEN: Because I wanted to know what it tasted like.

MOM: Well, what did it taste like?

STEPHEN: It tasted terrible. Why does Daddy drink it all the time?

MOM: Why do you think?

STEPHEN: I know—it's because he can't stop, right?

MOM: Right. Do you want that to happen to you?

STEPHEN: No.

MOM: Do you think you want to taste it anymore?

STEPHEN: No. Never.

Chapter Six
What You Can Expect

When children reach adolescence, they begin to test their own values, and the values of others. This is normal adolescent rebellion. No matter how they've been brought up, they have to see what else the world has to offer, so they can make educated decisions about their lives.

Kids experiment in all areas of their lives. It's natural for even the best kids to experiment a little during adolescence. A teenager who has been coached in saying no to drugs—both licit and illicit—will probably be able to stay away from cigarettes, since cigarettes have no dramatic enjoyable physical effect. The effects of alcohol, on the other hand, are more tangible.

Take Joey: He has a strong personality, is from a loving and communicative family, and has had proper coaching in saying no. It is fantasy to imagine that Joey will go through his adolescence without drinking alcohol several times—or even trying pot a few times. Surveys show that between fifty and sixty percent of high school seniors in 1985 have tried pot. More than likely, however, someone like Joey will experiment responsibly, and his or her experiments will go no further. Once Joey knows what it's like to be drunk, or high, he'll stop experimenting and settle into a pattern similar to that of his parents.

Children who are secure in saying no to the gateway drugs

have a set of reins that they can pull taut when their experimentation reaches the level of hard liquor or marijuana. But children who think nothing of drinking alcohol have nothing to hold them back from using harder drugs—and when a kid starts experimenting with crack, it's not experimentation anymore; it's a drug habit.

Studies show that drug use that begins during adolescence, while by no means good behavior, is far less dangerous than drug use that begins in pre-adolescence or post-adolescence. A nine-year-old with a drinking habit is much more of a cause for alarm than a fifteen-year-old with such a problem. Similarly, a twenty-five-year-old who begins drinking heavily is displaying signs of a deeper problem.

This does *not* mean that you should give your child the message that adolescent drug experimentation is expected, harmless behavior. It is your job to be the anchor for their value-testing. Their experimentation is *not* okay with you, and as long as they know that, it will shadow their actions. However, don't give them the "if I find out you've been drinking . . ." ultimatum, because that closes lines of communication. There's a fine line between disapproving of cigarettes and alcohol, and frightening your child to the point where he or she won't talk to you if there is a problem.

Chapter Seven
Stories for You and
Your Child

The rest of this book is devoted to stories for you to read with your children. Each story illustrates, in a way that a child can understand, the various topics addressed in the previous chapters.

Don't force your child to sit through all the stories in one or even two sittings. Read and discuss each story; continue reading only as long as your child seems interested. Use the questions at the end of the stories as springboards for conversations—explore your child's thoughts and feelings, and your own.

The children in these stories always do the right thing. Situations in the real world are not always so clear-cut, but proper coaching and good parent-child communication can make all the difference.

TAMMY'S STORY

There were a bunch of girls who smoked in the downstairs bathroom at school, but nine-year-old Tammy was new in school, and didn't know that. When she stepped into the bathroom to wash her hands, there were five girls there whom she knew from class. They were all smoking, and the room was full of smoke.

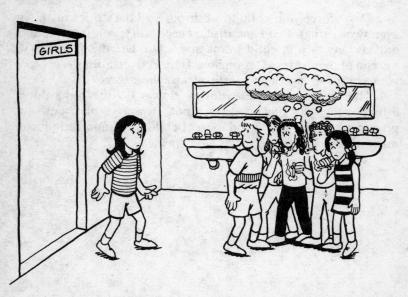

"Hi, Tammy," said Lisa, who was ten. "You want a smoke?"

"No," Tammy said, "I don't like cigarettes."

"Ever try one?" asked Lisa.

"No. I don't have to try something to know I don't like it."

"You want to be our friend, don't you?" asked one of the other girls.

"Yeah," said Tammy, "but not if I have to smoke. It smells terrible in here."

"C'mon, it's fun once you get used to it," the girl said.

"You're addicted to it!" Tammy said. "That's why you think it's fun."

"Huh?" said Lisa.

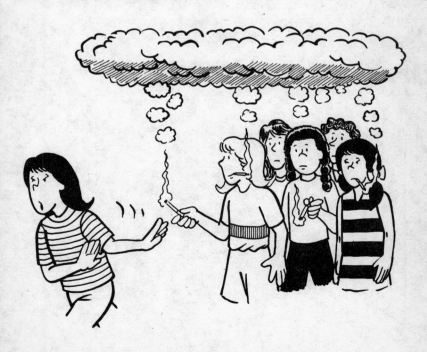

"That's right," said Tammy as Lisa took another drag on her cigarette. "Tobacco is a drug, and you're addicted."

"I'm not addicted," Lisa said. "I only smoke once or twice a week."

"Well, you should quit before it's too late!" Tammy said. She finished drying her hands and left, leaving the other girls to think about what she had said.

What else might Tammy have said to the girls about cigarettes?

BRAD'S STORY

Brad, who was seven, had to walk past a dark alley on the way home from school. "The Snakes" —the neighborhood's best known gang—hung out there.

One day the ball Brad was playing with rolled down the alley. He ran in to get it, and found

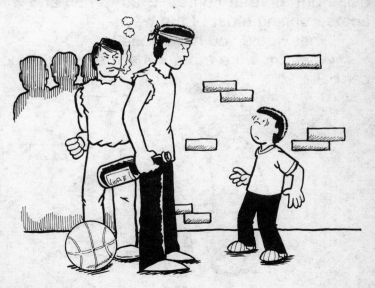

himself face to face with Bernie Muller, the leader of the Snakes. Bernie was much bigger than Brad, and very mean-looking. He picked up Brad's ball.

"Want your ball, kid?" Bernie asked.

"Yeah," said Brad.

Bernie held the ball out of reach, and with his other hand shoved a bottle of vodka at Brad. "Then you've got to drink this whole bottle!" The other kids in the alley laughed.

"No way," Brad said.

"Then you don't get your ball," said Bernie. Everyone laughed again. Bernie put the bottle in Brad's hand.

"C'mon," Bernie said, "you want to be cool like us, don't you?"

"No!" Brad answered. "Vodka isn't cool. It makes you forget stuff and gives you a head-ache!" He put the bottle down. "You can keep the ball, I got more at home." Brad turned and went home, running most of the way.

What would you have done?

What if it were a brand-new, expensive soc-cer ball?

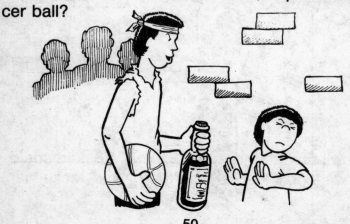

APRIL'S STORY

Ten-year-old April and her friend Jennifer were in the mall, looking at a mannequin in the window. The mannequin was slender and graceful, wearing very stylish clothes. April looked at her own reflection in the glass. She was a bit overweight. "I wonder if I'll ever be thin enough to wear something like that."

"You have to control your appetite," said Jennifer, who always thought she had all the answers.

"I've tried," said April. "I just can't. And I hate diets."

"Have you tried smoking?" asked Jennifer. "My sister smokes. She says smoking helped her control her appetite."

April thought about this. If she smoked she'd hurt her lungs, yellow her teeth, and make her

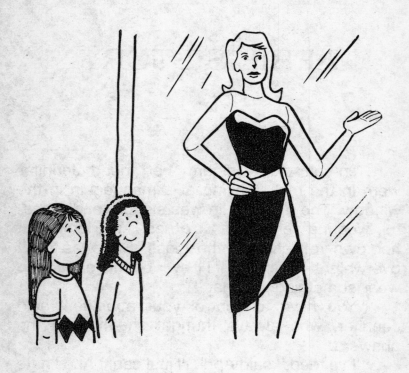

clothes smell bad. Besides, April knew lots of fat people who smoked. What Jennifer was saying just wasn't true.

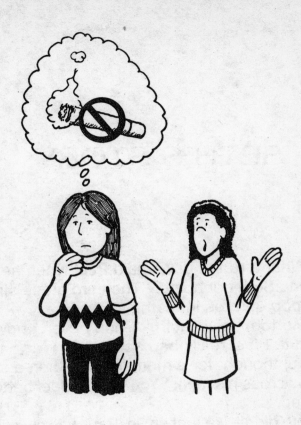

"I think I need to exercise more and eat less, that's all," April said. She didn't give smoking another thought.

Why do some people think smoking helps them lose weight?

SETH'S STORY

"What a rotten day," said Paul when he and his friend Seth got home. "The third grade stinks! I hate pop quizzes in math!"

"Me too," said Seth. "I don't even know if I passed it. I feel really bad about it."

Paul thought for a moment, and then a smile spread across his face. "You want to feel better?" he asked.

Seth didn't like that smile. Paul was always up to something no good when he smiled that way.

"Follow me," Paul said, leading Seth to a big wooden cabinet in the den. From the cabinet's bottom shelf, Paul pulled a little glass bottle that was almost full of a clear liquid. "Let's drink this stuff!"

"No," said Seth. "That's alcohol, and I'm not supposed to."

"No one'll know," said Paul. "C'mon, it tastes

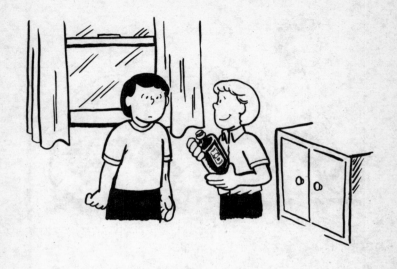

good. It's sweet and tastes like licorice." Paul dipped his pinky into the bottle, then stuck his finger in his mouth.

Seth said, "It doesn't taste good. You're just pretending it tastes good, because you think it's grown-up to like that stuff. It's not grown-up, it's stupid!"

"You're a baby!" Paul said.

Seth turned and headed for the front door. "I'm going home. I might feel bad about today's test, but I'll never feel bad enough to want to drink that stuff."

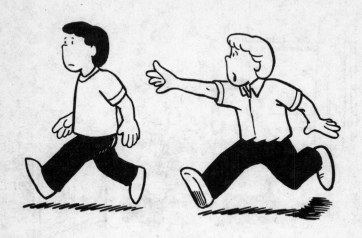

"Wait," shouted Paul, running after him, "I thought we were going to finish building my model plane today."

"Not unless you put that stuff away," Seth said.

Paul looked at the bottle in his hands, thought for a moment, then said, "Okay, I'll put it away."

"That's better," said Seth, smiling. Paul put the bottle away, and they went to his room to work on the model.

What would you have done if Paul didn't put the bottle away?

BRENDA'S STORY

Mitch was the best pitcher on his Little League team, and he thought all the girls in sixth grade had crushes on him—especially Brenda, who was very pretty. Brenda didn't like Mitch because he was so stuck up.

Mitch idolized professional baseball pitchers. He began to chew tobacco because he saw the pros doing it on television. Brenda could see an ugly bulge in one cheek, and brown spittle on his clothes.

There was going to be a big dance at school, and Mitch asked Brenda if she'd go with him. When he smiled she saw brown shreds of tobacco in his teeth.

"No way!" said Brenda, who always said exactly what she thought.

"Why not?" Mitch asked, shooting some tobacco spit out of the side of his mouth.

"Because you chew tobacco and you're gross!" Brenda said, and walked away. Mitch just stared after her.

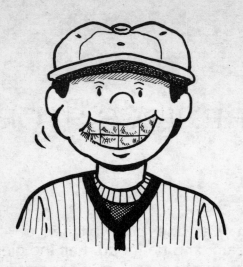

Later Brenda learned that no one would go to the dance with Mitch.

She hoped he would change his habits.

What would you tell Mitch about his tobacco-chewing habit?

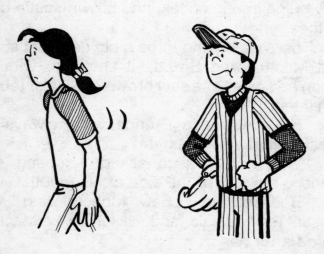

ROBBIE'S STORY

Robbie was at a party, and he felt pretty uncomfortable. Although he knew most of the kids there, nobody wanted to talk to him. Robbie had gotten to the party late, and it seemed like everyone else already had someone to talk to. Robbie just stood in a corner with his hands in his pockets, hoping someone would talk to him.

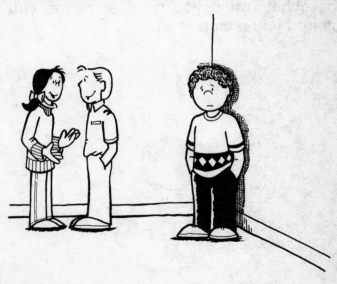

"You look silly with your hands in your pockets," said his friend Ben, coming over to him.

"Well, what should I do with my hands?" asked Robbie. "I feel dorky unless my hands are in my pockets."

"Here's what you do with your hands," Ben said. He grabbed Robbie's hand, putting a cigarette between two of his fingers. "Now you have something to do with your hands, and you look cool too!"

Robbie knew that there was no good reason to smoke, so he gave the cigarette back.

"I know something better to do with my hands," he said. Robbie went to the refrigerator, took out three apples, and began juggling. In a few minutes everyone was watching him, and when he finished, lots of people wanted to talk to him.

What would you do if someone you know offered you a cigarette?

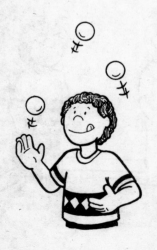

GEORGIA'S STORY

Ten-year-old Georgia had a sister named Cheryl. Cheryl was twenty, and a junior in college. Once while Cheryl was home for the holidays, Mom and Dad went away for a weekend and

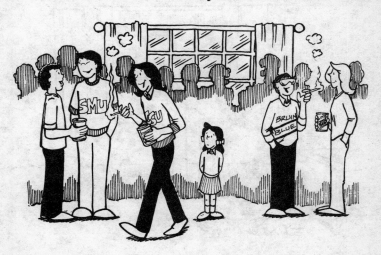

Cheryl threw a big party for all her friends. Cheryl let Georgia stay up late for the party. There was alcohol of all kinds and lots of people were smoking.

"You're getting to be a young lady now," Cheryl told Georgia. "If you don't tell Mom, you can have some wine."

"No, thanks," said Georgia.

"Oh! A goodie-two-shoes," said one of Cheryl's friends, laughing. Georgia ignored her. Pretty soon, people began to act silly, and one boy got sick, so Georgia went to her room.

When their parents came home in the morning, the house was a mess!

"Cheryl!" her father shouted. "What happened here?" Georgia saw Cheryl stumble out of her room holding her head as if it hurt to move.

"I just had a party," Cheryl said. "I feel awful!"

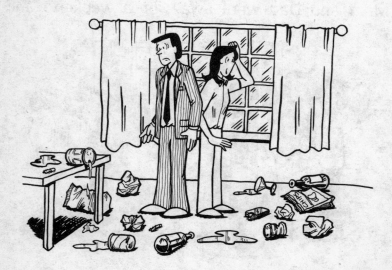

Georgia's mother shook her head. "How many times do you have to get sick before you learn not to get drunk?"

Cheryl didn't answer, and Georgia wondered if Cheryl would ever learn.

What would you tell Cheryl if she was your sister?

CAMERON'S STORY

Ever since they were little, Gary, Cameron's best friend, had tried to coax Cameron into doing things he shouldn't do. Now they were both ten, and Gary hadn't changed.

One day when they were bike riding, Gary saw a pack of cigarettes on the ground.

"Hey, let's smoke 'em!" said Gary.

"No way," said Cameron. "I don't want to get cancer."

Gary didn't listen. He picked up the pack, pulled out a cigarette, and tried to light it with some matches he was carrying.

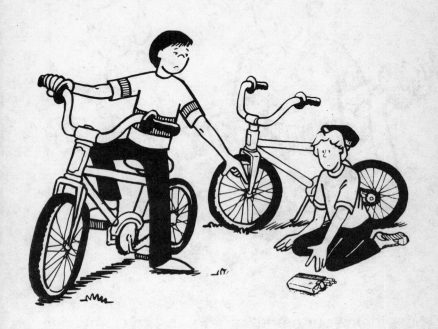

Thinking quickly, Cameron said, "Race you to the park!"

"Not now! I'm trying to light this cigarette," Cameron said.

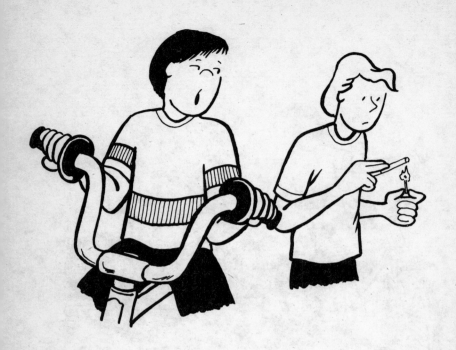

"On your mark!"
"Wait a second!"
"Get set!"
"I don't wanna race!"
"Go!" Cameron pedaled off quickly. Gary, who would never forfeit a race, dropped the cigarettes and rode after Cameron. In a minute he forgot completely about the cigarettes.

How else could Cameron have gotten Gary away from the cigarettes?

ANNA'S STORY

"I can quit smoking whenever I want to!" yelled thirteen-year-old Eddie. He was having another fight about smoking with his eight-year-old sister.

"Oh yeah?" said Anna. "I'll bet you ten dollars you can't quit for a month!"

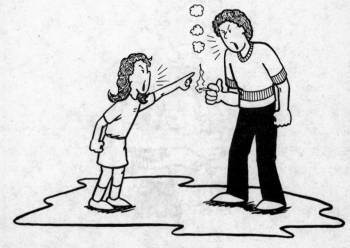

"Fine," said Eddie, shaking her hand. "It's a bet!"

Two weeks later, Anna caught Eddie sneaking a smoke behind the house.

"Fine!" said Eddie. "You win. I'll give you ten dollars."

"I don't want ten dollars," she said, almost crying. "I just want to help you quit smoking."

"I don't need help," said Eddie. "I can quit whenever I want to."

"Who do you think you're fooling, Eddie?" asked Anna.

Eddie looked down. "All right. I admit it. I can't stop. I want to, but I need help."

Anna gave him a big hug. "I love you," she said. "Let's go talk to Dad. I know he can help you."

What would you do if your brother or sister smoked?

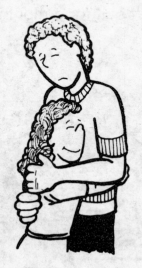

FRANKIE'S STORY

Frankie and Tina, both seven years old, were playing on the beach when a wave washed a bottle ashore.

"Hey, let's see if there's a message in the bottle!" said Tina. She pulled the bottle from the water to discover that it was half full of whiskey.

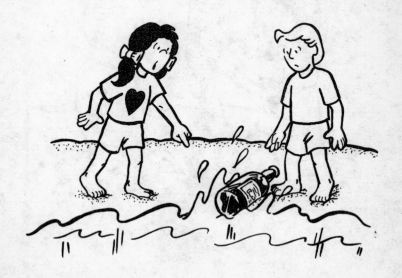

"Oh, wow!" Tina said, and a devious smile came over her face. "Let's try it!"

"Don't be dumb!" said Frankie. "The stuff's no good for you."

"Ah, you're no fun!"

"Being a drunk is no fun!" answered Frankie.

Tina began to think about her grandfather, who had died of a bad liver because he drank too much.

"You're right," said Tina, opening the bottle and pouring the whiskey into the sand. "Surf's up! Let's go in."

What would you do if you found a bottle of alcohol?

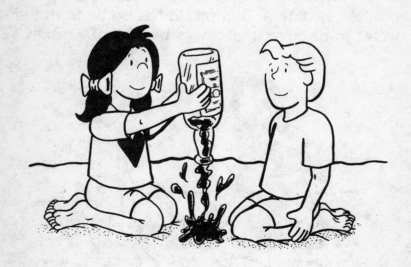

BARB'S STORY

Nine-year-old Barb ran into her friend Carrie on the way home from school; Carrie was waiting outside the supermarket.

"Hey, Barb," she called, "do you think you could lend me a dollar or two? I'll pay you back next week."

"Sure," said Barb, reaching for her purse. "What do you need it for?"

"My sister's in the store buying me something, and I have to pay her for it."

"What's she buying?" asked Barb.

"Cigarettes, that's all," Carrie answered.

"Cigarettes!" Barb said, wondering what kind of person would buy cigarettes for her nine-year-old sister. "Is that why you don't have any money left from your allowance? Did you spend it all on cigarettes?"

71

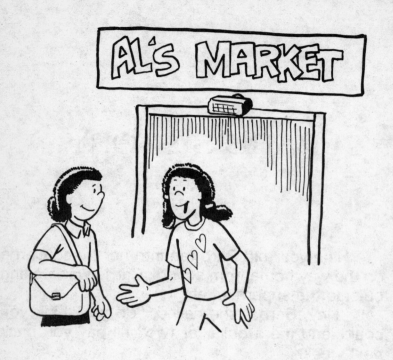

"Well, cigarettes are expensive," said Carrie. "Can I have the money?"

Barb closed her purse. "No way. I won't buy your cigarettes for you!"

"I thought you were my friend!" shouted Carrie.

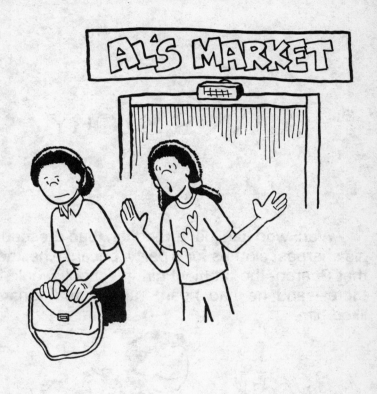

"I am," said Barb, "and that's why I won't help you poison your lungs."

What would you have said to Carrie?

ALAN'S STORY

Alan, who had just turned ten, had dressed in his sharpest clothes for a party, because he knew that Sharon, the prettiest girl in school, would be there—and he had heard rumors that Sharon liked him.

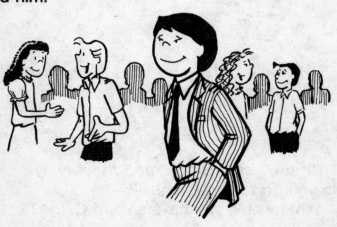

The party was crowded, and everyone was having a good time dancing. Alan was waiting for a chance to talk to Sharon. Finally, Sharon went outside, and Alan followed.

"Hi, Alan," she said when she saw him.

"Hi, Sharon. Good party, huh?"

"Yeah," she answered. Then she reached into her pocket and pulled out a pack of cigarettes.

"You smoke?" asked Alan. He couldn't believe it!

"Of course," she said. "Want one?"

"No thanks," Alan said. "Hey, why don't you come in and dance instead?"

"I'm tired of dancing," said Sharon. "What I need is a good smoke. Why don't you try one? You're old enough; you can smoke if you want to." Sharon took a long drag on her cigarette.

"But I *don't* want to."

Sharon laughed. "Maybe you're just a baby!"

"Sharon, why don't we just talk, and you can forget about smoking."

"No way," said Sharon. "I'll smoke whenever I want to."

"You mean you'd rather smoke by yourself than talk with someone?" asked Alan.

"That's right," said Sharon, puffing away.

Alan sighed. "See you around, then." Alan went back into the party, leaving Sharon to her cloud of smoke. She might have been pretty, thought Alan, but she was also pretty stupid.

What would you say to Sharon to stop her from smoking?

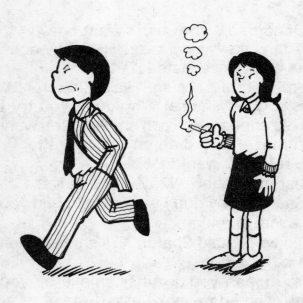

MARIA'S STORY

It was New Year's Eve, and Maria was at a party where everyone was celebrating.

Tanya held out a bottle of champagne to Maria, who was eight years old. "Happy New Year!" she yelled. "Drink some champagne!"

"No thanks," Maria said.

Tanya nudged Maria with her elbow. "C'mon, it's New Year's. I'm sure your parents won't mind. My parents let me!"

"No, I don't like the stuff."

Tanya eyed Maria for a moment like she was from another planet. "You're weird," said Tanya. "Fine, I'll drink the whole bottle myself!" And she did just that, and very quickly.

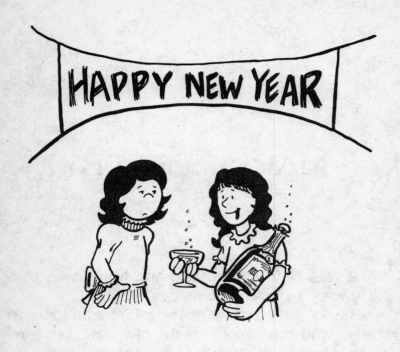

Soon Tanya was stumbling around. "Boy, do I feel drunk!" she said. She kept banging into things and laughing. She could barely stand up. Then the expression on her face changed.

"Tanya, are you okay?" asked Maria.

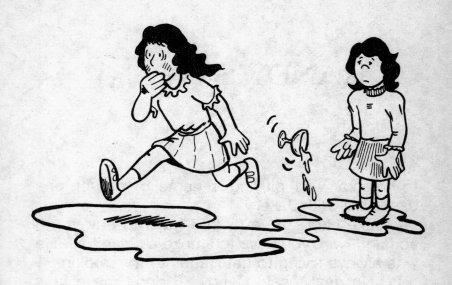

"I feel funny," said Tanya. Maria thought her friend looked green. In seconds Tanya ran into the bathroom, closed the door behind her, and was sick. By the sounds Tanya was making, Maria could tell Tanya was not having a happy New Year anymore.

What would you do if someone offered you a drink at a party?

RANDY'S STORY

Randy was playing a game of one-on-one basketball with Jake.

Jake said, "If you win, I have to buy you a soda. If I win, you have to smoke a cigarette." He was always trying to get Randy to try smoking.

"No deal," said Randy. "I don't make bets like that."

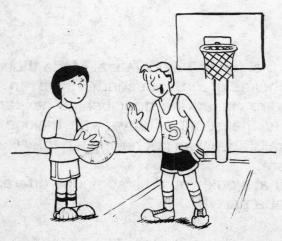

"Why not? It's fair."

"Nothing will get me to smoke a cigarette, not even a bet. How about if I buy you a soda too if you win?"

"Either you smoke a cigarette, or nothing," said Jake, putting his hands on his hips and waiting for Randy to decide.

"You're just trying to trick me into smoking!" said Randy.

"What's the big deal?" asked Jake. "It's just a bet. Are you afraid to make a bet, wimp?"

"No . . ." said Randy, "but I won't smoke." Randy took his basketball, and began to walk away.

"Chicken! Wimp! Baby!" screamed Jake, but Randy didn't care. He knew better.

What would you have done?

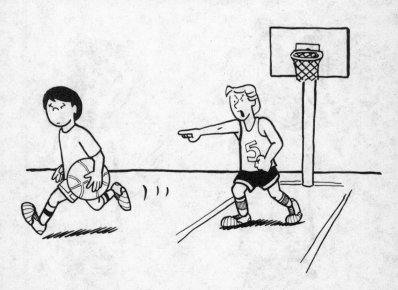

KIM'S STORY

Laurie was the fastest nine-year-old on the swim team. Kim was second fastest. She always worked hard, trying to beat Laurie, but she never could . . . and then Laurie began to smoke.

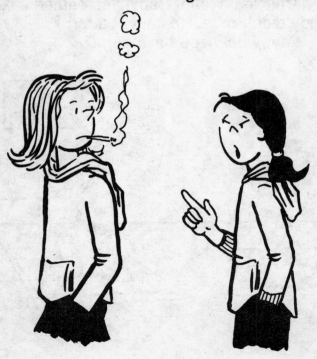

"You know, Laurie," said Kim, "smoking makes it hard for you to breathe when you swim."

"I don't believe that," said Laurie. "Smoking doesn't *really* hurt your lungs."

Finally the big meet of the year came. Laurie and Kim were both in the same event: the 50-yard freestyle sprint. When the gun went off, Kim dove in and swam the two-lap race with all her strength, as fast as she could. When she touched the pool wall at the end of the race, she was thrilled to find out that she had won! Then she saw that, two lanes away, Laurie was just finishing. Laurie grabbed onto the side of the pool, breathing heavily and coughing every few seconds.

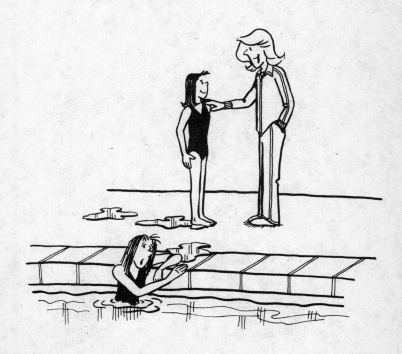

Later the coach congratulated Kim, then went up to Laurie. "You know, Laurie," said the coach, "your times are getting slower and slower every time you swim. What's the matter?"

Laurie didn't say anything, but Kim knew what the matter was.

Why couldn't Laurie swim fast anymore?

JOSÉ'S STORY

José didn't know what went on in the back of the school bus in the morning. The bus driver spent a lot of time yelling at the kids in the back, but he didn't seem to care what they did as long as they were quiet. Eight-year-old José, who usually sat in the front of the bus, decided, out of curiosity, to sit in the back.

"Hey, José," said Steve, who was sitting in the corner of the very last seat, "here, take one of these. Don't tell anyone." Steve handed José a miniature bottle of rum. Everyone in the back of the bus was sneaking sips from little bottles.

"Do you guys do this all the time?" asked José.

"Yeah," said Tara, who was sitting next to Steve. "It mellows us out before a hard day at school." She giggled and took a sip from her bottle.

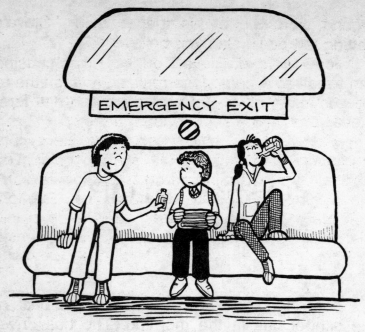

Now José knew why Steve, Tara, and some of the other kids were almost flunking out of school. With alcohol in their brains, how could they learn anything?

"Forget it," said José, giving back the bottle.

José began to walk to the front of the bus. Behind him, he heard Steve say, "You'll be in trouble if you tell anyone about this!"

José sat down in his usual place. He had said no, the way he knew he was supposed to, but he wanted to tell someone about what he'd seen. He didn't know if he should—Steve might come after him, or whoever he told might not believe him.

At first he didn't say anything, just stayed away from those kids, but a few weeks later, he saw Steve in the principal's office. José asked around, and one of his friends said, "Steve's getting left back! Can you believe it?"

José felt bad. Steve's drinking was causing him to fail at school. José realized it was time to tell someone, so he told the principal that Tara, Steve, and the others had been drinking.

The next day at the bus stop, Steve confronted José. "I'll teach you to tell the principal on us!" said Steve, and he swung at José. José didn't like to fight, but he had to defend himself. The fight didn't last very long, because Steve was drunk. His reflexes were slow, and he wasn't seeing straight. José, who was half his size, knocked him down in no time.

"I should have told someone sooner," said José. "If I did you might not have gotten left back. You shouldn't be mad at me, you should be mad at yourself."

Would you have told if you were José?

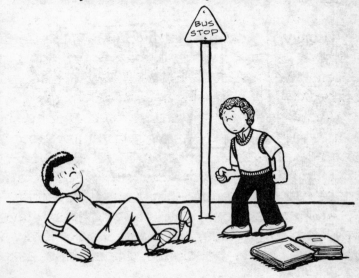

SANDRA'S STORY

Sandra was finally ten years old. Now she was old enough to be in the special club that all her friends belonged to.

Everyone was gathered in the treehouse. When Sandra climbed in, she was shocked to see that everyone there had a cigarette.

"So this is what they do secretly in the

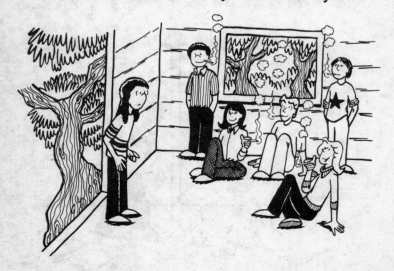

treehouse," she thought. Annie handed Sandra a cigarette.

"You have to smoke if you're going to be in our club. It's part of the rules," Annie said.

Sandra took the cigarette and broke it in half. "I won't smoke for anybody!" she said. "I don't care if you are my best friend."

"Well, I guess I'm not your best friend any more," said Annie, with a nasty look on her face.

"I guess not," Sandra said, and she left the treehouse. In no time at all Sandra found a whole new group of friends who didn't smoke.

What would you do if your best friend tried to make you smoke?

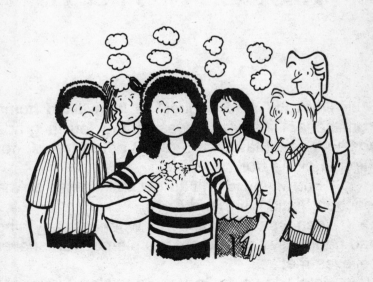

MIGUEL'S STORY

"Darn it!" said Miguel, as he walked home from school. "I wish I was in the fourth grade again. At least last year I didn't get in trouble for things I didn't do!"

"I know you didn't throw the eraser at the teacher," said his friend Cory.

"Yeah," said Miguel, "but whenever anything bad happens, I always get the blame—she never believes me!"

"Calm down," Cory said. "Here, I've got something that will relax you."

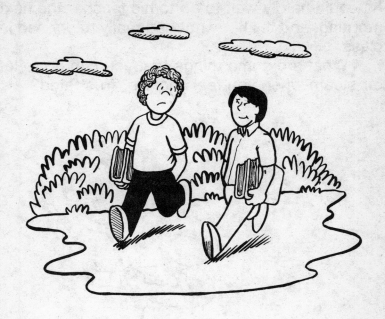

Cory reached into his pocket, and pulled out a flask of scotch. "Drink enough of this and your troubles will fly away," he said.

"That's not true," Miguel said. "That stuff will give me more problems."

Cory shrugged, and put the flask away.

When Miguel got home, he still felt frustrated and angry, so he got his tennis racket and went to the park. There, he practiced his tennis, hitting a ball against the handball wall for about half an hour, as hard as he could. When he was done, he didn't feel angry anymore. In fact, he felt so calm, he could hardly wait to go to his teacher the next morning, and tell her what had really happened in class.

What are some things that you can do to let off steam when you feel angry or frustrated?

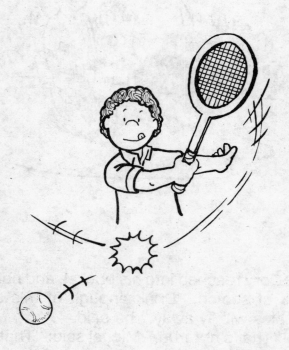

LYNETTE'S STORY

At Lynette's brother's wedding, almost everyone was drinking alcohol. Even the kids managed to get some.

"This is a rum and Coke," said her cousin Billy, who was eight years old, just like Lynette. "My dad said I could try it—you want some too?"

"Naah," said Lynette, "I don't want to become an alcoholic."

"Don't be stupid," said Billy. "You won't become an alcoholic if you take one drink."

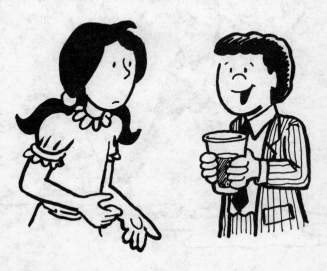

Lynette thought about it. She'd always trusted Billy before—then she saw Billy's dad. Uncle Rick was on the dance floor, acting crazy. He had a drink in one hand, and was staggering around and bumping into people. Lynette knew he had been drinking all night. Some people thought his stumbling was funny—but Lynette didn't. She thought it was sad.

"Look at your dad," said Lynette. "If that's what alcohol does to you, I don't want any. I don't want to look foolish."

Billy looked at his father. "He does look kind of dumb, doesn't he?" Billy put the rum and Coke on the table. "Let's get plain old Cokes," he said. "I like it better that way anyway."

What would you have done?

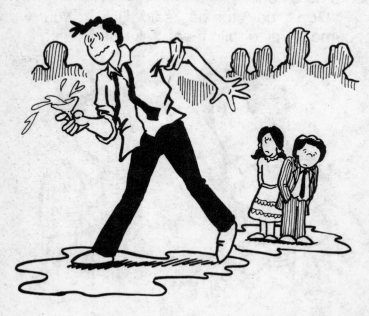

GORDIE'S STORY

At the state fair, eight-year-old Gordie and his seven-year-old cousin, Sammy, came across a flashy-looking tobacco-spitting booth.

"Come on, everyone's welcome," said the

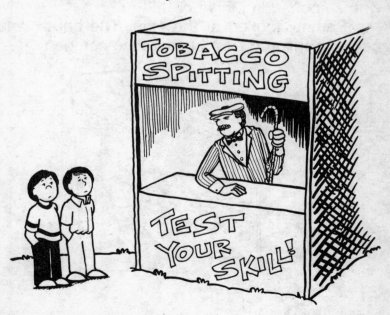

man in the booth. "Test your skill in tobacco-spitting. The furthest spit wins a prize!"

"Hey, let's try this," said Sammy. He stepped up to the counter.

"Well, my young friends," the man said, "step right up. Here's some tobacco for you." The man handed Sammy and Gordie each a bit of tobacco. "Chew it," he said, "it tastes good." Then he smiled, and the boys saw that his teeth were yellow-brown. He turned away a little and spat some tobacco juice onto the ground.

"Sammy, we'd better not," Gordie said. "You don't want your teeth to look like that, do you?"

"Well, I'm only going to do it once," said Sammy.

"But that's how you get hooked on it. Look who's sponsoring this booth!"

Sammy looked at the sign. The booth was being sponsored by a big tobacco company.

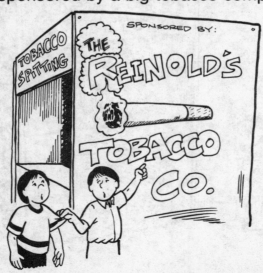

"Don't you see," said Gordie, "this is how that company gets kids to buy tobacco—they let kids try it for free, and before long they go out and buy it themselves. No thanks!" He dropped the tobacco onto the counter.

Sammy thought for a moment, then handed his tobacco back to the man.

"Oh well," the man said. "Next time, maybe."

"Probably not," said Gordie, as he and Sammy walked away.

What would you do?

JEANNIE'S STORY

One afternoon nine-year-old Jeannie passed a supermarket with her friends David, Kathy, and Pete. The door swung open, and out ran Larry, another of Jeannie's friends, along with a bunch of kids Jeannie knew from school. Jeannie didn't like those kids very much, because they always got into trouble.

"Guess what we did," Larry said. He opened his jacket, and showed the kids two bottles he was hiding underneath. "We just stole some beer," he whispered.

"Larry!" said Jeannie. "You're not allowed to drink beer!"

"Says who!" Larry began to walk off with his new friends.

"Larry, I thought you were our friend!" Jeannie said.

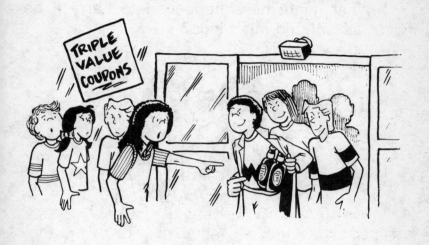

Larry turned to face her. "Well, I am, but can't I be their friend too?"

"Not if it means you're going to steal beer. Either you're their friend or you're our friend, because our friends don't steal beer," said Jeannie.

"Well, are you coming?" called Ricky, one of Larry's new friends.

Larry thought for a moment, then turned to Ricky and said, "Naah, I just remembered, I got homework to do. See you later."

Ricky and his friends left with their stolen beer.

"I'm glad you know who your *real* friends are," said Jeannie. Larry put down his beers, and they all ran off to play.

How can you stop your friends from doing bad things?

What might have happened to Larry if he went off with the other kids?

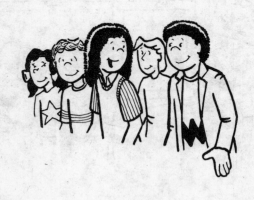

ZACK'S STORY

One day eight-year-old Zack went to the movies with his friend Perry. Ten minutes into the movie, a group of kids sat down in front of them. They were loud, obnoxious, and made fun of the movie. Zack could smell that they had been drinking alcohol. Perry began to giggle at the other kids' behavior.

"I don't like these kids," Zack said. "Let's change our seats."

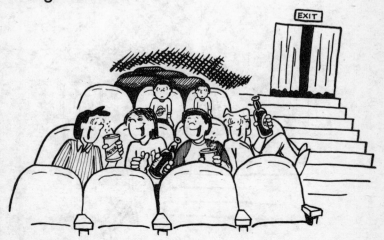

"Don't you think they're funny?" asked Perry.

"No," said Zack. "They're drunk, and they're acting stupid."

Zack got up and Perry followed. They moved to seats across the theater.

Ten minutes later Perry tapped Zack on the shoulder and said, "Hey, look, the usher's throwing those kids out of the theater!"

Zack turned to watch the rowdy kids stumbling up the aisle. "That's what happens when you get drunk," said Zack. "You get loud and act silly, and get thrown out of places."

Soon the kids were out of the theater and everyone else seemed a lot happier.

What would you do if kids like that sat near you in a movie theater, or anyplace else?

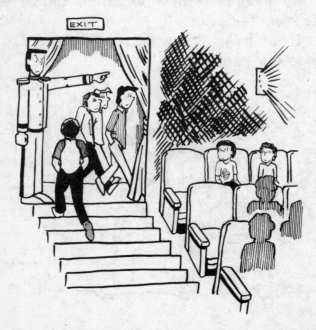

AUDREY'S STORY

One hot summer afternoon, eight-year-old Audrey sat on the beach with her thirteen-year-old sister Teri, getting a tan. Teri was puffing on cigarettes and looking at the boys.

"Wow, look at him!" said Teri, pointing to a tall muscular boy who was walking along the

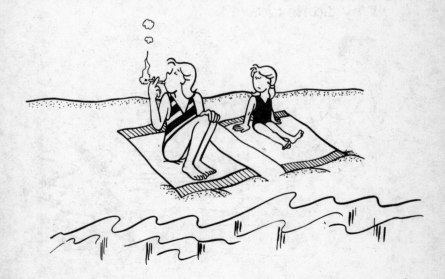

beach. Teri smiled at him. The boy smiled back, and began to walk towards them.

"He's coming this way," said Teri. She put out her cigarette in the sand, and fixed up her hair. Audrey watched as the boy came closer.

"Hi," said the boy, kneeling down. "My name is Rex."

"I'm Teri. Nice to meet you."

Rex's smile disappeared. He pulled back about a foot and began waving his hand in front of his face.

"Gross!" he said. "Your breath smells like a wet ashtray!" He stood up and walked away just as quickly as he came. "Bye."

Audrey thought this was very funny, and began laughing hysterically.

"Oh shut up!" said Teri. She looked very angry.

Why did Rex leave?

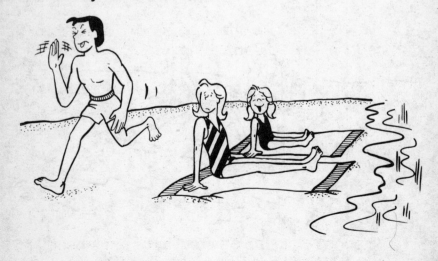

NOAH'S STORY

On the fifth rainy day in a row, during Easter vacation, Noah was sitting in a friend's basement with other kids.

"This is boring," said Kevin. "What can we do?"

"I know! Let's go drink some beer," said Joe.

"Yeah," added Jan, "there's nothing else to do."

"What do you mean there's nothing else to do? We can play basketball at the gym," said Noah.

"Boring!" said the others.

"We could go to a movie," suggested Noah.

"Boring," said the others.

"We could play board games. What about that?"

"Boring," said the others. "Let's drink beer."

Noah stood up. "You know what? You guys

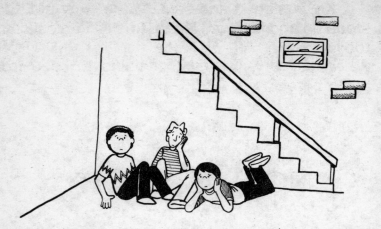

are just addicted to boredom. You don't know how to make your own fun. I wonder what you'll be addicted to next."

The kids looked at each other and thought about what Noah had said.

"I don't know about you," said Noah, "but I'm going to the movies." Noah began to climb the stairs.

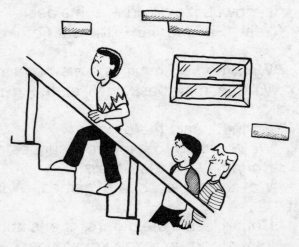

Kevin sighed and said, "Sure, why not." He stood up and followed Noah. And all the rest came too.

What can you think of doing to keep from being bored?

ALLIE'S STORY

Allie was studying at Lisa's house, because they had a big test coming up. When Lisa's mom went out, Lisa reached into her pocket and pulled out a pack of cigarettes. She lit one.

"You shouldn't be smoking. It can kill you," said Allie.

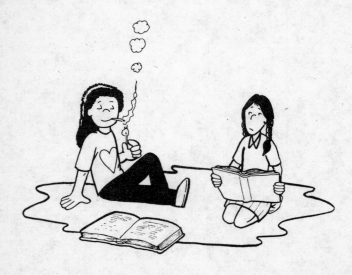

"Don't worry about it," said Lisa, blowing smoke in Allie's face. Allie began to cough.

"You're making me choke; can't you please stop?" asked Allie.

"No! This is my house, I have a right to smoke here," Lisa said, puffing away.

"Fine," said Allie, "and I have a right to breathe." Allie stood up, taking her books. "I'll find some friends who aren't so inconsiderate," she said as she left.

What would you do?

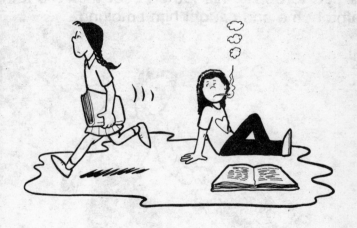

RYAN'S STORY

Ryan's dad smoked two packs of cigarettes a day. One day when Ryan was alone, he tried to smoke a cigarette. He coughed a lot and it tasted terrible, but he finished the cigarette, because he wanted to be like his father. Just then his father came home and caught him smoking.

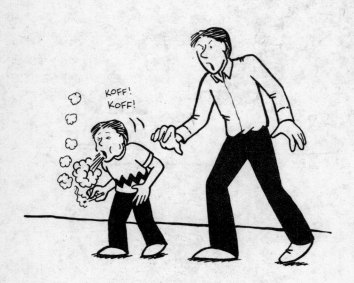

"What are you, crazy?" yelled his dad. "You'll ruin your lungs. Don't ever do that again!"

"But you do it," Ryan said. "Why can't I?"

Ryan's dad thought for a moment. He sat down with Ryan so they could talk.

"I don't want to smoke," said Ryan's dad.

"Then why do you?"

"Because I can't stop. I wish I never started. I was stupid to start smoking. I don't want you to be stupid too." Ryan's dad leaned back. He smiled a little. "When *I* was seven years old I was just like you; I could run twice around the block and not even feel tired. Now if I run even to the corner, I start coughing and can't catch my breath. Smoking ruined my lungs. Do you want that to happen to you?"

Ryan looked down. "No."

"Then stop wondering what it's like to smoke," said his dad, " 'cause I can tell you what it's like. It's lousy." And then he started to cough.

What would you say to your dad if you were Ryan?

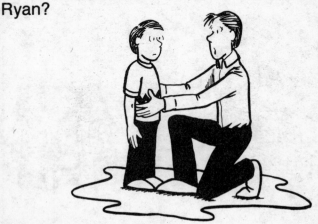

JUANITA'S STORY

Juanita was at the video arcade with her friend Rita. As she finished a game, Juanita saw that Rita had gone over to the other side of the arcade and was talking with some other kids they

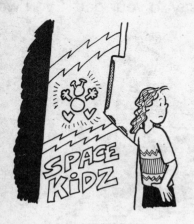 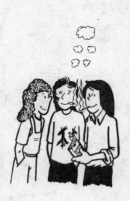

both knew from school. Juanita knew that those kids smoked. In a few seconds one of them had pulled out a pack of cigarettes and offered one to Rita. At first Rita shook her head no, but they put it into her hand, and finally Rita took it.

"Hey, Rita," called Juanita. "Let's play a video game together—my treat."

Rita gave the girl back her cigarette and ran over to Juanita. Juanita put two of her quarters into the game machine.

"Thanks for the game, Juanita," Rita said.

"It's the least I could do to keep you away from cigarettes," answered Juanita.

What would you do to keep a friend away from cigarettes or alcohol?

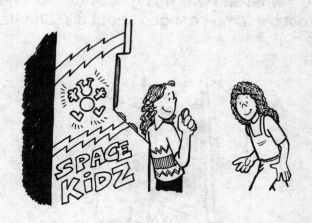

LEE'S STORY

One day after school, Lee, age seven, caught his eleven-year-old sister, Jill, sneaking drinks from their parents' liquor cabinet.

"You have to promise not to tell Mom and Dad," she told Lee.

"Okay," Lee said. At first he thought she knew what she was doing . . . but soon, he began to notice some changes about Jill. She had been

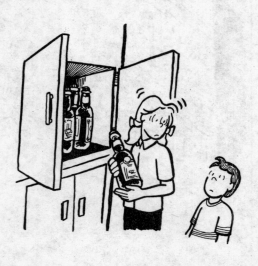

waking up later—and with terrible headaches. She was also beginning to forget things. He was afraid to break his promise to Jill, but he knew that she was becoming an alcoholic.

Late one night, while Jill slept off all the alcohol she'd drunk, Lee told his parents all about it. He knew he had broken his promise, but he was too worried about Jill to keep that promise.

If your brother or sister began drinking, what would you do?

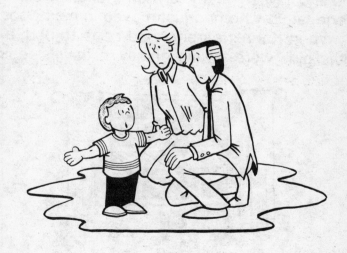

KARIN'S STORY

Karin had a slumber party for her ninth birthday, and invited many of her friends, including Valerie, a girl who had just moved in next door.

When Karin's parents had gone to bed, and all the girls were talking quietly in their sleeping

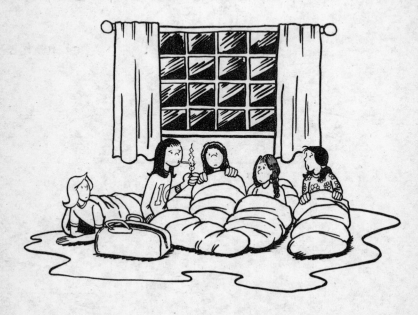

bags, Karin saw the flash of a match: Valerie had lit up a cigarette!

"Ooh! Look, Valerie's smoking," said one of the girls.

"Can I try one?" asked Laura.

"Sure," Valerie said, handing out cigarettes. Then she pulled a big bottle of scotch from her overnight bag. "It's my mom's," she said, "but she doesn't care if I drink it."

Karin knew she shouldn't let this go on, but she didn't know how to stop it. Valerie took a drink from the bottle in between drags on the cigarette.

"Don't!" said Karin. "There's no smoking allowed in my house! My parents will smell it!"

"No they won't," said Valerie. Laura lit her cigarette too.

"Put those out now!" Karin said firmly. They all looked at Karin, then put their cigarettes out—except for Valerie.

"Karin's right," said Dorie. "It's her house, and we shouldn't be smoking anyway."

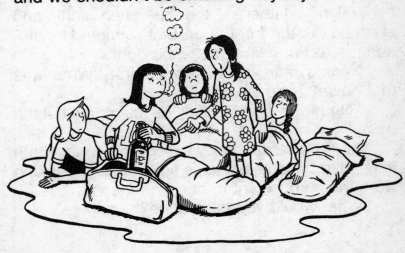

"Put that bottle away too," said Karin. "This is a slumber party, not a drug party."

"These aren't drugs!" said Valerie.

"Shows how much you know!" said Karin.

Valerie shrugged. She wasn't really listening. She kept smoking and drinking. Karin decided she had to make a stand.

"Stop it now, or else!" she said.

"Or else what?"

"Or else I'll throw you out of my house!"

Valerie laughed. "Don't be ridiculous!"

"I mean it!"

Valerie looked around at the other girls. "Are we gonna let her do this to us?" The other girls didn't answer; they just stared. "You can't make me leave!" said Valerie.

"Oh yeah?" Karin went to the table and picked up the phone. "I'm calling your mom."

Valerie's eyes grew wide, and Karin knew she had won. "Fine!" Valerie said. "I'll leave! I don't want to be seen with you anyway!"

Valerie gathered together her stuff and stormed out the front door. She slammed it hard, and ran to her own house next door.

Karin's mom came downstairs. "What was that noise?" she asked.

"Nothing," said Dorie. "We just threw out the trash."

All the girls laughed, except for Karin. Karin felt bad for Valerie, because smoking and drinking were more important to her than friends.

What would you have done?

KEN'S STORY

It was the biggest game of the season, and everyone on the team was ready to play their best . . . that is, *almost* everyone.

Eleven-year-old Ken had seen his best friend, Blake, arrive just as the game started. Ken didn't think anything was wrong until it was Blake's turn to bat.

It was the first inning, no outs, and Ken's team had three men on base. Blake was up.

"Knock it out of the ballpark!" said Ken as Blake passed him in the dugout.

"You bet I will," Blake said. His words were sort of slurred, and Ken could smell alcohol on his breath. Ken began to worry.

"Blake," he asked, "have you been drinking alcohol?"

"Don't worry," said Blake. "It makes me

relaxed, so I can play better." Blake picked up his bat, and headed for home plate.

"Batter up!" yelled the umpire, and Blake took his position. The pitcher threw three perfect pitches, but each time, Blake swung late, and missed.

"You're out!" yelled the ump. Everyone was amazed, because Blake was the best hitter on the team. Blake dropped his bat in anger, and staggered toward the dugout, then stumbled and fell to one knee. Ken ran out and helped him up, and together they went to the dugout.

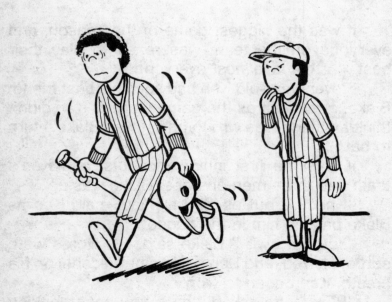

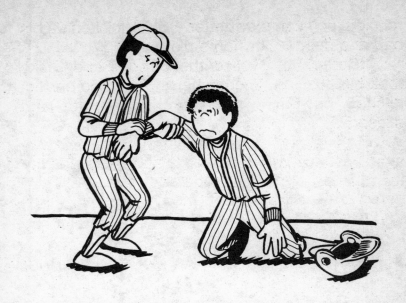

"I don't feel so good," Blake said, with his head in his hands.

"Maybe you should tell the coach what you did," suggested Ken.

"But he'll yell at me!"

"Don't worry," said Ken, "I'll go with you."

Together they told the coach what Blake had done. The coach was more worried than angry. He made arrangements to talk with Blake after the game. Blake couldn't play for the rest of the day, because his reflexes were too slow, and without Blake, the team wasn't able to win. Both Ken and Blake were disappointed, but they had both learned a valuable lesson.

What else might you need fast reflexes for?

If you started drinking alcohol, who would you be letting down?